Table of Contents

Chapter 1. – Introduction to this guide

Whether you are getting a tooth extracted or undergoing open heart surgery, it is perfectly common to have some apprehension. Though the doctor's office probably provides you with pamphlets, the words on the pages often feel stale and distant. Wouldn't it be nice to hear a casual, first-hand experience?

Be forewarned that this handbook contains honesty of many different sorts. Helpful honesty. Comical honesty. Repulsive honesty. In my opinion, honesty is important. Not just with others, but also with ourselves, which is often the hardest.

Sometimes we need a pal to help us get over an obstacle or through a difficult time. Our medical professionals often only have time to explain the main gist of the surgery process, and sometimes we need a bit more detail on what to expect.

You may have pondered, "What can I expect while at the hospital? How do I prepare for the thoughts and emotions prior to and after the surgery?" This casual guide contains my personal experiences, and it is meant to provide practical tips and to inspire looking through a playful/whimsical lens.

Doctors can't always pinpoint the [correct] diagnosis right away. It is up to the patient to find ways of maintaining a healthy mindset throughout the entire process. I have gone "doctor-hopping" for two **completely** different issues because they couldn't figure out what the problem was, and that took a toll. Physically, mentally, and emotionally.

Some patients will be ready for their surgery, and others will pretend they are ready, put on a smile, and try to hide their distress.

Which method is correct? Both.

I became intrigued by the research I came across which proved that mindset and physical mannerisms can in fact alter our feelings. Studies have proven that if you smile for an extended period of time, your brain will actually begin to feel happy. There are many things in life we take for granted and should be grateful for, yet somehow, we often tend to focus on the few negative aspects and current fears. There is nothing wrong with having fears or worries, but I invite you to become aware of them and then work towards conquering them.

These days, my main fear is standing in line and not knowing if I'll be ready to order when I get to the counter. If you're familiar with New York deli culture, you know what I mean.

The way my eyes perceived the sky

However, it wasn't long ago that my fear of hospitals and surgeries loomed above me like the dark skies during a heavy thunderstorm. Even when the sun was shining, my world appeared dull. It seemed like my life was ending.

It wasn't the way life actually *was*; I was viewing it through layers of lenses that I had created in my mind.

The way the sky probably looked

It's certainly not a habit I exhibited before; I had always been optimistic, busy with violin lessons, vocal training, and dance practice.

I don't recall my first surgery -- adenoid removal. I was a young child at the time. I don't recall my first set of stitches -- mall accident.

The first surgery that I *do* remember came after fifteen months of limping on an ankle that I had injured during dance practice. Needless to say, that surgery was *warmly* welcomed.

It is with that request for recovery, and that hankering for healing that I pushed through the physical therapy. It was important to remind myself that it was painful yet needed, and that the journey will either make me stronger or weaker, depending on how I decide to tackle each day.

If *only* I had the same pre-game in my mind before my thyroid surgery. Well, I decided to shift my thoughts so that I would. It became important to take things one day at a time, and love each chapter for whatever it brings.

Much like a book, our lives are divided into chapter. Not every chapter is easy or exciting. However, each chapter shapes us. The things we go through make us *us*. We grow, we learn, and we can then help others by sharing our personal experiences.

The original social media posts that I made during my Total Thyroidectomy Pre-Op and Post-Op are featured in pink, and they are examples of the positive thought practices that are suggested in this guidebook.

Please note: This guidebook is not meant to diagnose or treat any illness. It is not meant to replace medical advice; it is meant to inspire your mental and emotional preparation so that you can journey on with tranquility and strength.

Chapter 2. - The weeks and hours prior

Let's begin with a multiple-choice question. You have just been told you need surgery. What is your immediate reaction?

a.   Your mind begins racing and you cannot stop thinking ahead into the vast unknown

b.   You crap your pants [Hopefully figuratively, but no judging here]

c.   You sit, blinking your eyes and reaching for carbs and chocolate to reduce the anxiety

Based on your answer, you may have also just figured out whether you are predominately analytical, dismal, or basically just an emotional eater. I'm kidding; I'm no expert on personality tests. If you've never taken one, though, I recommend it so that you may better understand how your mind operates.

When shocking situations emerge that we didn't expect in our ideal life plan, we reflexively jump to label them 'scary' or 'bad'. Sometimes we feel like the world is going to end, and then we look back years later in appreciation for the new path it had redirected us to. For some reason, many people are eager - and sometimes willing to risk their lives - to undergo cosmetic procedures, but are afraid and nervous when they have a health-related surgery ahead of them.

It is understandable, of course, that when a physical issue pops up out of nowhere, thoughts begin to race. Unfortunately, in many cases the shock factor has lead to emotional issues, including:

- Anxiety

- Depression

- Stress

- Anger

- Fear

You'll probably experience a roller coaster of emotions. It's okay to not be okay. However, it's unhealthy to remain 'not okay' for extended periods of time. Years of research lead me to believe in the importance of mindfulness and counteracting toxic stress.

There is a correlation between high levels of anxiety/stress and chronic issues. The 'fight or flight' response that your body generates is unhealthy if maintained for lengthy periods. The last we need is for one issue to invite further illness. Stressful events can trigger an increase in heart rate and blood pressure, and high stress often contributes to a weakened immune system, a change in eating habits, and a change in sleeping patterns.

Since the length of your diagnosis-to-recovery journey is unknown, it is helpful to utilize a method that can maintain your inner peace.

Several weeks of unrelenting pain due to an ankle injury during dance rehearsal led me to make an appointment with a doctor to figure out what was wrong. I explained that there was a loud pop, and I had experienced pain ever since. The x-rays did not show anything worrisome, according to her, and she then told me it was all in my head. Needless to say, I switched doctors.

One year and three months later: finally, after half a dozen different tests I had never heard of (up until that point I had only known of x-rays,) it was determined that although the bone wasn't fractured, there was cartilage floating within my ankle joint. They found the culprit, and I required a simple surgery to remove those fragments.

No wonder walking around my high school halls had become so difficult. It felt great to learn that there was indeed a reason for my excruciating pain and inability to perform regular daily activities, and yet it was frightening to hear that it would take months of physical therapy to regain strength and normal function. The immense pain I felt every time I limped around was enough of a reason to get the surgery done as soon as possible. I was exuberant at the idea of being able to stand up and put my weight on both feet.

Now, here is an example of the opposite:

A few years later, I had seen a handful of specialists to find out why I was losing my voice. During a yearly physical, my general practitioner noticed a large nodule on my thyroid gland and immediately referred me to an Endocrinologist. That quickly led to ultrasounds, biopsies, and blood tests that showed that my thyroid antibodies were extremely high. The ultrasounds proved that there were *numerous* nodules, and that they were rubbing against my vocal cords, causing my voice to go in and out randomly. Furthermore, the abnormal thyroid tissue was a scare because the doctors warned me of the dangers of keeping a gland that seems to be cancerous. The verdict was that the entire thyroid had to be removed as soon as possible. In fact, my surgeon's schedule was completely full, so he scheduled an emergency operation on the upcoming Saturday.

Talk about shock. There was virtually no time to process all this new information. Even though I had been through surgery before, I had massive anxiety about this operation and the effects it may have. I had to resign from the performing job I had at the time, and was therefore unemployed. My career would be halted, and the doctor didn't know whether my vocal cords would ever recover or not. Cue the tears. I wished that I were not single because I was *sure* men would run away from my eerily-slit throat. Cue *more* tears.

After a couple days of being sad, worried, and upset about my life's current circumstances and the mere assumptions of what was to come, I realized that I needed to change my mentality. It was time for a complete makeover of the spirit. It takes hard work to change gloom into positivity, but it is worth every ounce of effort. There are others who are in more pain than you are. There are others who aren't able to find a diagnosis at all. Offer assistance to someone who may need some. Volunteer at homeless shelter if you are able to. It may take your mind off your worries.

"Life's a test, right? So hopefully my good deeds are earning me some extra credit points :)"

Posted on April 20th

Instead of pessimistically assuming that you will be in a huge amount of pain, have excessive stiffness, and/or that the surgery may leave unsightly scarring, focus on the positive. In what ways will this operation help you? Remind yourself that you are beautiful, inside and out, and this minor bump in the road is intended to make you healthier. Optimism is key. So is humor.

Loving yourself is essential to the healing process. Many people do not realize that the healing process can be launched long before the surgery date. The healing process begins the moment you start read this guidebook!

The goal of the process is to put you at ease and allow your body and mind to unite. Health is multi-faceted. Do you exercise and eat a nutritious, balanced diet? Strength is important, and it's important to note that there is physical and emotional strength.

The emotional aspect is equally in need of extra attention during this time in comparison to previous daily life. Pamper yourself; nourish your mind and body with food, faith, and happy thoughts.

Depending on how much time you have between the day you found out you needed surgery and the scheduled surgery day, you can plan accordingly.

Make a list of 20 things you are grateful for. Do something you have been wanting to do. Visit a restaurant you have been wanting to try. Go out into the sunshine. Get your hair cut. Watch some of your favorite feel-good movies. Watch something funny. Laugh. Eat healthy foods. Dance. Make funny faces in the mirror. Laugh more. Eat your favorite food. Enjoy it and smile.

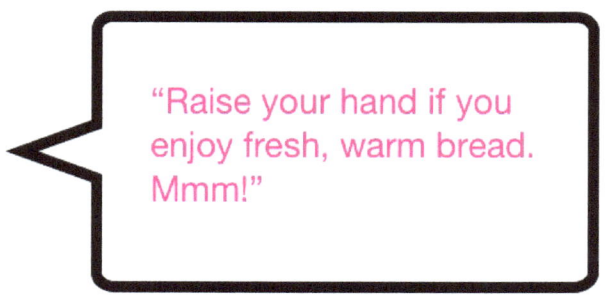

"Raise your hand if you enjoy fresh, warm bread. Mmm!"

Posted on April 21st

Consider giving your operation a name. It may help you see it in a different light and also make it sound much more awesome.

"Operation: drink milkshake when I wake up."

"Operation: eat chocolate covered strawberries afterwards."

See, doesn't that sound harmless and even *exciting*? If you answered no, then clearly you may want to insert *your* favorite food or drink instead. It allows you to visualize making it through the procedure and looking forward to the delectable goodies that await you.

Instead of food, perhaps try focusing on one of your goals, such as hiking one of the mountains you have yet to explore, or visiting a city or historic landmark you have been wanting to see. Have you been looking forward to signing up for a taekwondo class or a cooking class? There is a beauty in closing your eyes and seeing yourself doing these things; being there.

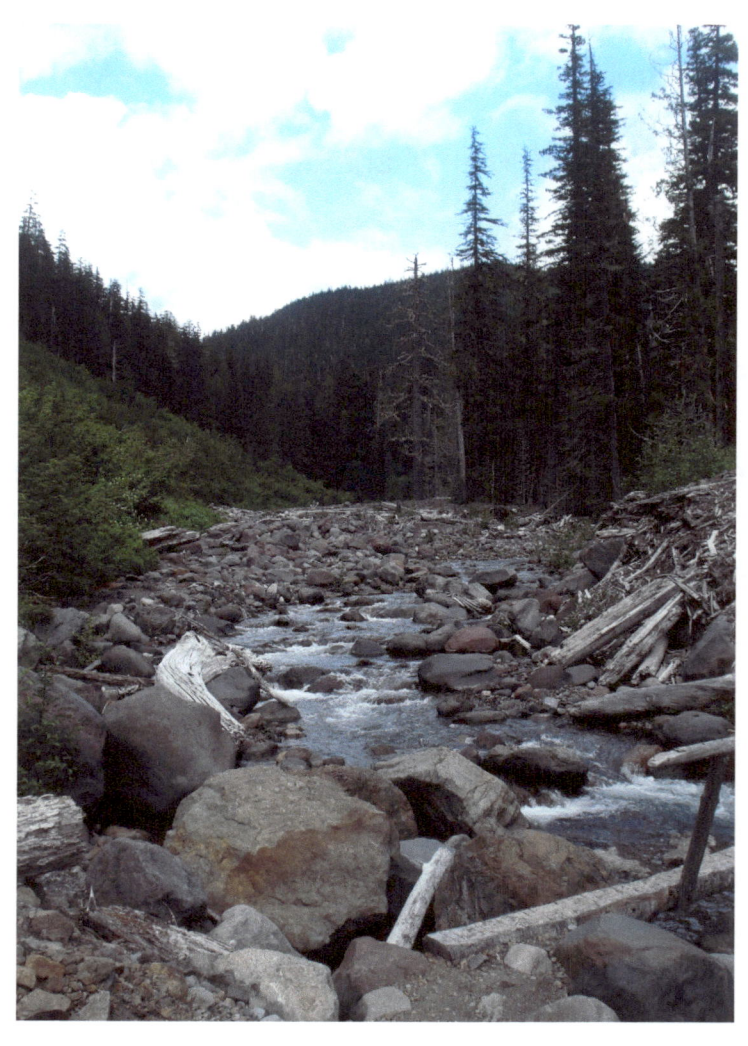

Photographed while hiking Mt. Rainier

Thoughts are incredibly powerful. That is why there is immense power in meditation and Law of Attraction. Tell yourself that your body will be better after the surgery. Imagine the body healing and making you feel rejuvenated.

Detoxing the body is commonly advised for health purposes. Detoxing the mind is just as needed. Remember, it's okay to have fear and worry prior to your surgery, but in order to begin healing from the inside out, you can begin transforming yourself from *anxious* to *prepared*.

Do you practice introspection? It is amazing what mindfulness, stillness, and drowning out noise can do. When we are alone with our thoughts, it meant to inspire contemplation and growth.

The body and the mind are connected. It is up to *us* to heal the way we *think*. Take time to reflect.

- Why are you getting this surgery?

- How has your current condition unpleasantly affected your daily life?

- Write down any pain you have had, and look back at it after your surgery because hopefully the pain - physical or emotional - will no longer exist. If you're not experiencing, perhaps your doctor suggested the surgery will benefit your body by allowing your system to run better.

- What *exactly* are you worried about?

- In what ways could your life be *improved* by this surgery?

- Are you maintaining healthy eating habits?

- Are you maintaining healthy sleeping patterns?

- Will you feel better if you relinquish control and put your trust in what you most   strongly believe in: God/The Universe/Science?

- Do you have enough **balance** in your life? (hobbies, friends, family, work, and thoughts about this illness/ surgery)

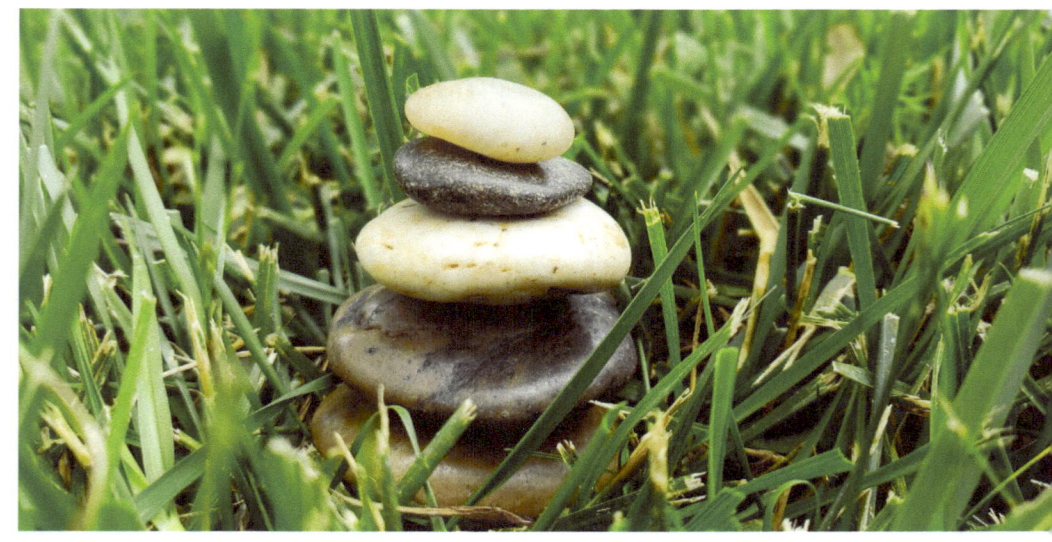

Meditating while balancing rocks

Consider utilizing this visualization meditation to stimulate a mind-body connection:

Close your eyes. Breathe slowly/deeply/consciously. Focus on your inhalations and exhalations. Make a conscious effort to make your inhalations and exhalations the same length. Picture things in your life that have made you happy. People/pets/places/material objects. Relax your body; get rid of physical tension from your shoulders, back, arms, and legs. Ask yourself why you are nervous about the surgery. Why do you have these worries? After you confront each fear, visualize the opposite. Picture the surgery going well, and picture your healing going well. Visualize yourself in the near future at the height of full health. Picture yourself achieving your biggest goal in life. As you inhale deeply, see your prospects blooming larger and larger. Exhale, sending your positivity out to great distances. State who you are and what you are going to become. Next, take a deep inhalation, hold your breath for a few seconds, inhale again to stretch the lungs further, then exhale loudly. Repeat the following a few times: "My body is strong. It can handle this. My mind is strong. I can handle this. I am strong. I am healthy."

Have you ever cut your finger and noticed how quickly the skin rebuilds? The reality is that the body has a natural ability to heal itself on a microscopic level. A great thing to remember is that the body repairs itself during deep sleep. Good sleep is crucial because organs and muscles get their needed recovery time, and the immune system gets a boost. Are you familiar with the "Sleeping Beauty" story? Give yourself the liberty of being a "Healing Cutie" by listening to your body and giving it the rest it needs. It would be fun to slip on an eye mask, turn to someone, and say, "Healing process activated" in a robot voice.

Aside from mental and emotional preparations for your surgery, you will want to pack a bag containing items you may need and/or want. You should feel as comfortable as possible during your hospital stay. Some good items include a toothbrush, toothpaste, phone charger, lotion, lip balm, breath mints, favorite plush toy, favorite music, and some extra party hats. Bring something colorful! Bring something that takes you to your happy place, like a framed photograph or collage of favorite photos. Consider bringing some coloring books and crayons, or you can bring crossword puzzles and mad-libs. How about some glow-in-the-dark toys? Is there a specific theme you have in mind? Don't hesitate to plan. After all, it's *your* party.

Oh, and for those who would rather maximize their relaxation time rather than party, pack your sleep mask and play some spa music!

Chapter 3. - What to wear: how to look and feel your best

Ah, the big day has arrived. You're ready for this. In fact, you probably already packed your special bag of items the night before!

It's time to get dressed! Just like any big event, it's all about how you look. On top of that, it's about how you *feel*. The goal of all your preparations leading up to this day was to put yourself at ease. Consider dressing in a simple outfit that is easy to get into and out of. You will want to be comfortable when entering and leaving the hospital. Besides, you are going to end up changing into a lovely hospital gown. When tied correctly, it can do wonderful things for your figure. Gala-goers would be jealous. You'll have some time to experiment with various styles.

Once you enter the Pre-Operative area, you'll fill out paperwork, verify your identity, and get prepped by the nurses. Do you have any last-minute questions? This is a great time to ask! You will be given a wristband with all your information. Double check that the information on the wristband is correct [and is *yours*.]

You'll be provided with a hospital gown and possibly a hair cap (AKA slumber party hat #1.) Next, it will be time to climb onto that fun bed with wheels, where they start your IV and attempt to keep you calm. You're not scared of needles, right? If so, they'll give you something *verrrryyy* special to help your anxiety…

Chapter 4. - Happy juice and anesthesia

Surprise! The anesthesiologist will dash in through a curtain and introduce himself/ herself. It would be ten times more fun if they would burst into song and dance, but alas, they must give you the boring spiel about the upcoming rituals.

You may first be given what is known as "happy juice" to calm your nerves, and then once they wheel you to the operating room, you will be administered some **crazy gas** - refer back to this as reference #1.

You may not remember getting wheeled into the operating room after having received the "happy juice," and you should definitely take that as a positive sign. It is a good indication that you won't be awake when they start doing their chicken dance. That's probably not part of their operating procedure, but it is funny to imagine.

You will usually be monitored in order to ensure that you stay asleep during the entire operation. The anesthesia has a tendency to make people loopy.

Caution: you will probably utter nonsensical foolishness...unknowingly, of course.

When the hospital staff ask you questions, you are likely to say regrettable things. They will either laugh it off or send you to counseling.

Hopefully they will just nod and smile, and soon after you'll drift off into sleep.

Gooood niiiight!

* Further pondering: They really ought to consider taking full advantage of the anesthesia once it is administered. Think of all the other procedures we could combine with this one! Why not bring in someone to thread eyebrows and wax upper lips/other sensitive areas? Why not perform surgeries *and* liposuction while a patient is knocked out and unable to feel the stinging?! I'm sure many patients would appreciate a two-for-one special!

Chapter 5. - ?!@%*#!!?!

Neither words nor random computer keyboard characters can describe the immediate confusion and panic that ensue when waking up in the recovery room. You will probably still be loopy, and you may be in and out of sleep for several minutes.

My suggestion: speak with caution. Anything you say may be used against you...

The good news is that you may feel extremely refreshed once you wake up. In my case, I felt like I had been asleep for a week. That anesthesia certainly put the 'slumber' in 'slumber party'.

It is difficult for me to remember what conversations occurred during my stay in the recovery area, but nothing distressing comes to mind. None of the staff mentioned any embarrassing uttering. That's a good sign, right?

You may experience dry mouth, chapped lips, and/or coughing, but do not be alarmed. The nurses will keep track of your progress to make sure nothing unusual happens.

It won't be long before you get wheeled out of the recovery room and into your very own space the hospital. This will be your special quarters during your stay, and the location of your very own slumber party!

"Raise your hand if you like watching funny movies in your hospital room :)"

Posted on April 23rd

Chapter 6. – Nurses vs. Visitors

You will not be alone during your hospital stay! Even if your friends or family are not able to swing by, be assured that there are extremely kind nurses who are specially trained in postoperative units to help guide you through the recovery process. Don't worry; they are going to be at your side when you need something. All you have to do is press a button and someone leaps into the room!

Having family, friends, and visitors you know *personally* will brighten up your day and be great additions to your slumber party. If they come empty-handed, however, you should make them feel guilty and ask for extra gifts on your birthday or favorite holiday.

Try to remember that this phase doesn't have to be all about *you* and your medical issues. It might help if you take your mind off your current situation. For example, talk to other patients; wish them well. Ask your nurses about their favorite movies, favorite food, dream vacation, etc. Strike up conversation, be genuine, and be friendly.

Perhaps you can go on a scavenger hunt around the halls! Can you find a nurse with green shoes? Do you see a yellow mug anywhere? How many pens can you spot at the nurses station?

If you find yourself bored at night or in need of a daily constitutional, you can do what I did:

"My IV drip stand and I go on short walks together. We have a real connection."

Posted on April 23rd

Another time, one of the female nurses who looked after me joined me for a walk up and down the hall. It was late during the night, and she was able to spare about fifteen minutes to take a stroll and chit chat with me (and my IV drip stand, which was rolling along next to me.) It felt like I made a new friend, and it felt like I had invited her into my world — my slumber party. She was intrigued by this glimpse into my world.

I implore you to invent methods of having an enjoyable hospital stay, as keeping yourself entertained - or at least happy - is essential to your slumber party. Every person who walks into your hospital room is joining in on whatever spontaneous activity that is going on. They will hold your hand and lend an ear. They can even help you get out of bed when you need to use the restroom. How sweet is that?! You can tell them some cheesy jokes as a way of thanking them. They will be glad to have you as a patient, especially if you also treat them kindly as they continue to take care of you. Whether your stay is one night or several nights, nurses and lab technicians will love the gratitude you show them.

In the case of my Thyroidectomy, the length of my hospital stay was dependent on the calcium levels in my blood. I ended up staying longer than initially anticipated. The lab technicians came in to draw blood out of the same arm every six hours and boy, did it drive me crazy waiting to hear those results. I desperately wanted the painful vampire lab people to stop draining my veins, but I knew that it was vital for my health. Therefore, I again shifted my frame of mind. It became a long comedy sketch.

"Lab lady said, "You bruise easily? Your vein is black/blue." I said, "Well 4 other lab ppl drilled in the same spot & took blood from me!"

Posted on April 24th

That would explain it, right? Sure, my arm felt like it was nearly going to fall off, however, every time they drew my blood, and every time the nurses came to give me pills and check on me, I thanked them and smiled. During those moments of pain, my "thank you" may have only been a whisper, but I was certain that they understood my appreciation. I was grateful for their assistance and their surprise visits to my slumber party.

Chapter 7. - Intestinal Ridiculousness

Once you are given the green light to start eating and/ or drinking, take it slowly - if you can stop yourself from devouring everything at the speed of light - because although you woke up from the surgery, your intestines may still be asleep. Remember reference #1? That was the fun type of gas.

Now I will teach you about the second reference to crazy gas.

It seems the only type of gas society deems as appropriate to discuss is the type used to fuel the vehicles we drive. In some countries, the other type is not as taboo. It is crucial to speak of gas and bowel movements with your doctors and nurses because it gives an insight to your general health. Yes, folks...not only does the gas we emit *smell*, but it also *speaks* volumes.

Since certain painkillers can aggravate the bloating and constipation, it is important to let your doctors and nurses know what you are feeling every step of the way.

A more recognized feeling will develop eventually, and if you are anything like me you will start craving detailed cuisine. Your stomach may soon launch rumbling and begin begging for food, and that might distract you from your distended abdomen.

"...Hopefully I'll be allowed to eat in a few hours- that's one of my favorite pastimes."

Posted on April 23rd

Hospital food can be quite tasty, especially when you have not had anything to eat or drink in a looooong time (usually 8 hours before surgery.)

You will be given a list of food you are allowed to eat, so you just order what sounds appetizing and take note of what you would order again for your next meal or snack.

The applesauce tasted delicious and kept calling my name for two days in a row, so I ordered that a handful of times with other dishes.

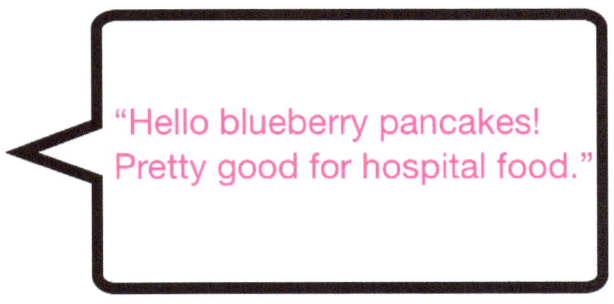

"Hello blueberry pancakes! Pretty good for hospital food."

Posted on April 24th

It may take a couple days before your bowels move, and it is not a comfortable feeling.

If it takes longer than that or if you are experiencing severe bloating and extreme pain, you should call your doctor right away. Do not feel embarrassed. It is important to discuss this type of gas with your healthcare professionals.

Chapter 8. - Relax; Allow yourself to heal

Take the journey one hour at a time, and allow yourself time to visualize a healthier, happier you. The key word here is *allow*.

"...Let's hope the next blood test includes better results so that I can go home."

Posted on April 24th

Often times, we get so caught up in work or catching up on things we missed while in the hospital. Remember to get enough sleep so that your body can repair itself further. Breathe, pace yourself, and allow healing thoughts to continue flowing.

"Yay I can leave the hospital after my calcium level gets back to normal :)"

Posted on April 24th

After my thyroid surgery, the hardest things for me to temporarily give up were the driver's seat of my car, yoga, and hiking. However, looking back, I am grateful that I could even *do* those things again after my ankle injury.

Once you have been given the 'green light' to leave the hospital, you may be given specific instructions, extra bandages/medical tools, and prescriptions - either temporary or long-term. You may also want to consider seeking nutrition counseling, as there may be natural supplements and/or new diet plans that could benefit you.

Following your hospital discharge, you may need follow-up visits with your doctor and/or additional treatment, such as physical therapy or speech therapy.

There may be scars and scar tissue, and while it can become easy to focus on the pain or looks, you could instead see it as part of your 'slumber party memory book'. Look beyond the scars, as others will too. Do not allow the scars to make you feel less beautiful. Or less *anything*. You can continue making the best of every situation. Love yourself!

Follow your doctor's specific instructions regarding what you can and cannot do during the first few weeks after surgery in order to allow your body to fully heal properly and completely. You would not want to undo what the surgeon has mended. As tempting as it may be, if you are not allowed to jog, please do not jog. If you are not allowed to lift anything heavy, please find someone to help you.

Deep breathing, meditation, and visualization exercises remain an important part of the recovery phase. Maintain healthy eating habits and get enough of that healing deep sleep. Do you enjoy yoga? There are certain poses that can promote organ healing.

Even if the healing phase takes longer than you had hoped it would, try your best to remain positive. Perhaps you are being taken on this path for a reason. Where ever life leads you, meet it with the least amount of resistance and anger as possible. Remain open to what the world hands you next, and find your own way of maintaining serenity.

Let your strength surprise you. You **can** handle this.

"Strenuous hike in the mountains? Check. Relaxing lunch on the beach? Check. ...Dolphins near the shore?! Exciting surprise! Lovely day!"

Posted on June 2nd

At the beginning of this new chapter of your life, allow the challenges to inspire further personal growth. My ankle surgery, followed by months of painful physical therapy, pushed me to grow as a person. Health is the fusion of internal and external factors. You can improve your body's function by seeking additional health-related knowledge and maintaining a positive mindset and approach to life.

Consider keeping a journal to monitor how the medicines, treatments, foods, exercises, etc. make you feel. Keeping a journal will also aid in your reflection. It is a great way to track your mental, emotional, and physical growth after the operation.

Do you still have that list of 20 things you are grateful for? Read through it again. Try adding a few more things to that list.

If you ever feel alone in your journey, or you find that your family and/or friends don't quite understand, please seek 1-on-1 therapy and/or a support group near you. It may benefit you to interact with others who have had this particular surgery, illness, or trauma. There are many emotional advantages of having someone to talk to about the journey, and you may also be able to inspire someone else's views on the healing process!

Begin the process of getting over the knife before you even enter the operating room, and after the operation, continue visualization exercises.

Live each of your chapters to the fullest. Encourage full healing to blossom within you by maintaining optimism, strength, and serenity - with a dash of playfulness, of course. You are a healing cutie.

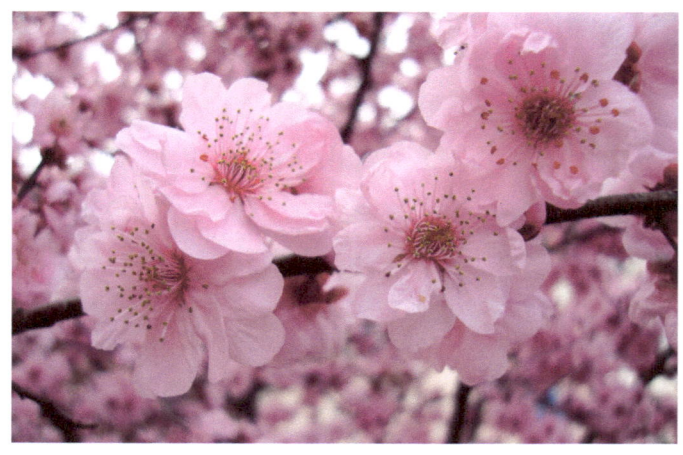

Visualize your healing as a blooming flower

P.S. - Wishing you a fun and healthy slumber party!